Discover the Mediterranean Lifestyle

Share the Healthy Mediterranean Diet with Someone Special

Sasha Merianelli

Table of Contents

Blueberry Pudding Cake

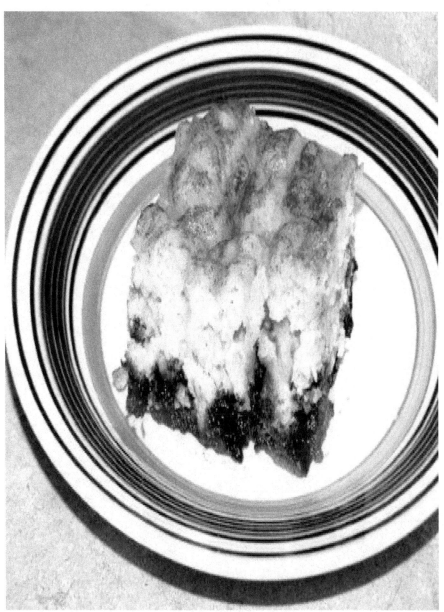

Preparation time:

15 minutes Cooking time: 25 minutes Servings: 6

Ingredients:

- 3 cups blueberries
- 3/4 cup sugar, divided
- tablespoon freshly squeezed lemon juice 6 tablespoons unsalted butter, softened
- teaspoons pure vanilla extract
- 1 teaspoon freshly grated lemon zest 1 egg white
- 11/2 teaspoons sodium-free baking powder 2 tablespoons low-fat milk
- 2/3 cup white whole-wheat flour

Directions:

1. Preheat oven to 400°F. Oiled an 8-inch square baking pan lightly with oil and set aside. Place blueberries into a mixing bowl. Add 1/4 cup sugar and the lemon juice and toss well to coat.

2. Pour berries into the prepared baking pan, place on the middle rack in the oven, and bake for 5 minutes. Remove from the oven and set aside. Place the butter and remaining 1/2 cup sugar into a mixing bowl and beat to combine.

3. Add the vanilla, lemon zest, and egg white and mix well. Add the baking powder and milk and stir. Gradually add in the flour, mixing until combined.

4. Pour batter over the cooked blueberries. Bake within 20 minutes, until golden brown. Serve warm or cool.

Nutrition: Calories: 300

Fat: 12 g

Protein: 2 g

Sodium: 14 mg

Fiber: 2 g

Carbohydrates: 46 g

Sugar: 32 g

Peanut Butter Banana Bread Bites

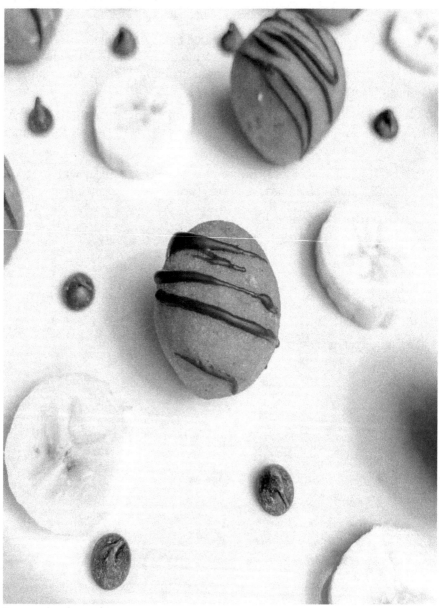

Preparation time:

10 minutes Cooking Time: 20 minutes Servings: 24

Ingredients:

- 1½ cups whole-wheat pastry flour 2 tablespoons ground flaxseed
- teaspoon baking powder
- ½ teaspoon kosher or sea salt
- ½ teaspoon ground cinnamon 3 ripe bananas, peeled
- large eggs
- 2 tablespoons canola oil
- ½ cup dark brown sugar 2 tablespoons honey
- ½ cup natural creamy peanut butter
- ¼ cup nonfat Greek yogurt 1 teaspoon vanilla extract
- ¼ cup unsalted roasted peanuts, crushed

Directions:

1. Preheat the oven to 350°F. Oiled a 24-cup mini muffin tin with cooking spray. In a bowl, whisk the flour, flaxseed, baking powder, salt, and cinnamon. Beat the bananas in a separate bowl with a hand mixer set on low.

2. Add the eggs, one at a time, then add the canola oil, brown sugar, and honey. Adjust the speed to medium and beat until fluffy. Add the peanut butter, Greek yogurt, and vanilla extract and mix until combined. Lower the speed to low, then beat in the dry ingredient mixture until just combined.

3. Put the mixture into each of the muffin wells about three-quarters of the way full. Tap it on the counter until the batter is evenly spread out.

4. Top with the crushed peanuts. Bake within 20 minutes, until a toothpick inserted into the center of a bite, comes out clean. Let rest on the counter until cooled. Remove the bites from the muffin tin. Serve.

Nutrition: Calories: 123

Fat: 5 g

Sodium: 81 mg

Carbs: 17 g

Fiber: 2 g

Sugar: 8 g

Protein: 3 g

Toasted Almond Ambrosia

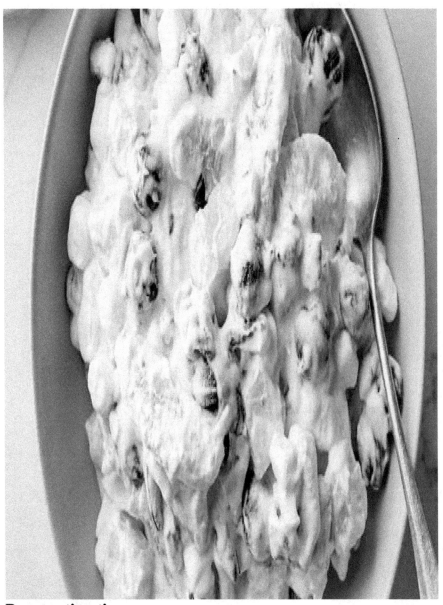

Preparation time:

10 minutes Cooking Time: 20 minutes Servings: 2

Ingredients:

- ½ Cup Almonds, Slivered

- ½ Cup Coconut, Shredded & Unsweetened 3 Cups Pineapple, Cubed

- 5 Oranges, Segment

- 2 Red Apples, Cored & Diced 2 Tablespoons Cream Sherry Mint Leaves, Fresh to Garnish

- Banana, Halved Lengthwise, Peeled & Sliced

Directions:

1. Start by heating your oven to 325, and then get out a baking sheet. Roast your almonds for ten minutes, making sure they're spread out evenly. Transfer them to a plate and then toast your coconut on the same baking sheet.

2. Toast for ten minutes. Mix your banana, sherry, oranges, apples, and pineapple in a bowl. Divide the mixture, not serving bowls and top with coconut and almonds. Garnish with mint before serving.

Nutrition: Calories: 177

Fat: 4.9 g

Sodium: 13 mg

Carbs: 36 g

Fiber: 0 g

Sugar: 0 g

Protein: 3.4 g

Apricot Biscotti

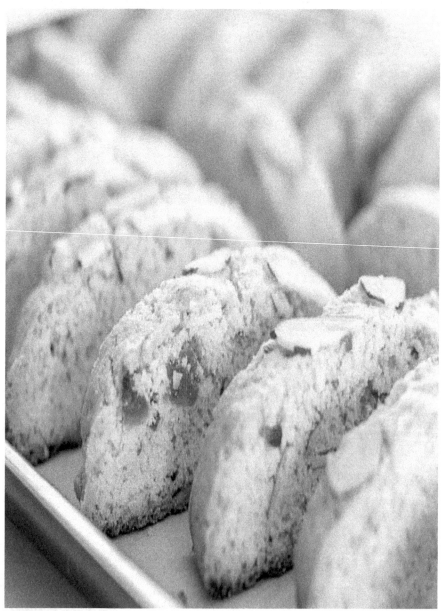

Preparation time:

10 minutes Cooking Time: 50 minutes Servings: 4

Ingredients:

- Tablespoons Honey, Dark 2 Tablespoons Olive Oil
- ½ Teaspoon Almond Extract
- ¼ Cup Almonds, Chopped Roughly 2/3 Cup Apricots, Dried
- 2 Tablespoons Milk, 1% & Low Fat
- 2 Eggs, Beaten Lightly
- ¾ Cup Whole Wheat Flour
- ¾ Cup All-Purpose Flour
- ¼ Cup Brown Sugar, Packed Firm 1 Teaspoon Baking Powder

Directions:

1. Start by heating the oven to 350, then mix your baking powder, brown sugar, and flours in a bowl. Whisk your canola oil, eggs, almond extract, honey, and milk. Mix until it forms a smooth dough. Fold in the apricots and almonds.

2. Put your dough on plastic wrap, and then roll it out to a twelve-inch-long and three-inch wide rectangle. Place this dough on a baking sheet, and bake for twenty-five minutes. It should turn golden brown. Allow it to cool, slice it into ½ inch thick slices, and then bake for another fifteen minutes. It should be crispy.

Nutrition: Calories: 291

Fat: 2 g

Sodium: 123 mg

Carbs: 12 g

Fiber: 0 g

Sugar: 0 g

Protein: 2 g

Apple & Berry Cobbler

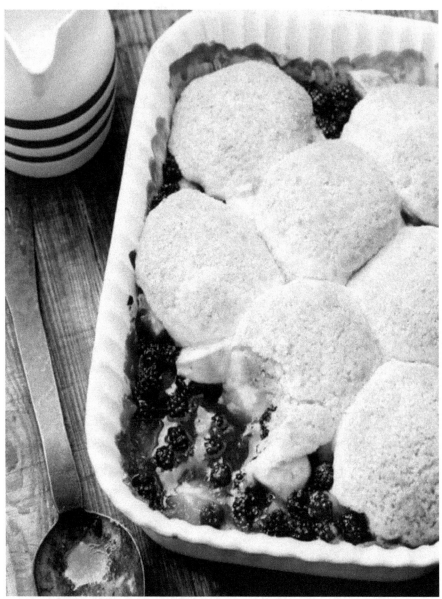

Preparation time:

10 minutes Cooking Time: 40 minutes Servings: 4

Ingredients:

Filling:

- Cup Blueberries, Fresh 2 Cups Apples, Chopped 1 Cup Raspberries, Fresh
- Tablespoons Brown Sugar 1 Teaspoon Lemon Zest
- 2 Teaspoon Lemon Juice, Fresh
- ½ Teaspoon Ground Cinnamon 1 ½ Tablespoons Corn Starch
- Topping:
- ¾ Cup Whole Wheat Pastry Flour 1 ½ Tablespoon Brown Sugar
- ½ Teaspoon Vanilla Extract, Pure
- ¼ Cup Soy Milk
- ¼ Teaspoon Sea Salt, Fine 1 Egg White

Directions:

1. Turn your oven to 350, and get out six small ramekins. Grease them with cooking spray. Mix your lemon juice, lemon zest, blueberries, sugar, cinnamon, raspberries, and apples in a bowl. Stir in your cornstarch, mixing until it dissolves.

2. Beat your egg white in a different bowl, whisking it with sugar, vanilla, soy milk, and pastry flour. Divide your berry mixture between the ramekins and top with the vanilla topping. Put your ramekins on a baking sheet, baking for thirty minutes. The top should be golden brown before serving.

Nutrition: Calories: 131

Fat: 0 g

Sodium: 14 mg

Carbs: 13.8 g

Fiber: 0 g

Sugar: 0 g

Protein: 7.2 g

Mixed Fruit Compote Cups

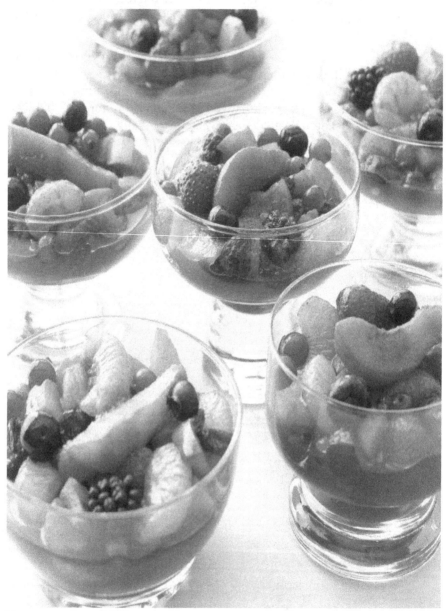

Preparation time:

5 minutes Cooking Time: 15 minutes Servings: 2

Ingredients:

- 1 ¼ Cup Water
- ½ Cup Orange juice
- 12 Ounces Mixed Dried Fruit 1 Teaspoon Ground Cinnamon
- ¼ Teaspoon Ground Ginger
- ¼ Teaspoon Ground Nutmeg
- 4 Cups Vanilla Frozen Yogurt, Fat-Free

Directions:

1. Mix your dried fruit, nutmeg, cinnamon, water, orange juice, and ginger in a saucepan. Cover, and allow it to cook over medium heat for ten minutes. Remove the cover and then cook for another ten minutes. Add your frozen yogurt to serving cups, and top with the fruit mixture.

Nutrition: Calories: 228

Fat: 5.7 g

Cholesterol: 15 mg

Sodium: 114 mg

Carbs: 12.4 g

Fiber: 0 g

Sugar: 0 g

Protein: 9.1 g

Cauliflower Breakfast Porridge

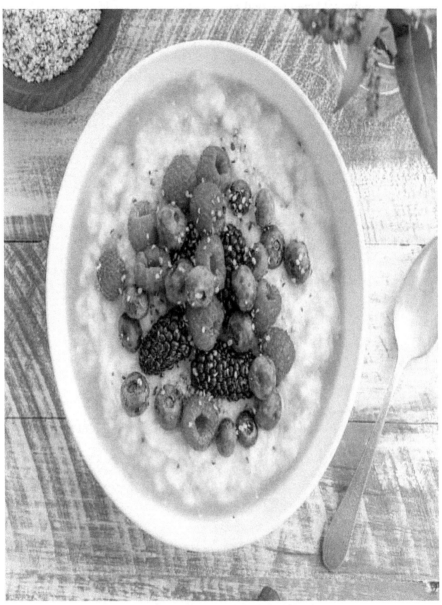

Prep time:

5 minutes | Cook time: 5 minutes | Serves 2

Ingredients

2 cups riced cauliflower

¾ cup unsweetened almond milk

4 tablespoons extra-virgin olive oil, divided

2 teaspoons grated fresh orange peel (from ½ orange)

½ teaspoon almond extract or vanilla extract

½ teaspoon ground cinnamon

⅛ teaspoon salt

4 tablespoons chopped walnuts, divided

1 to 2 teaspoons maple syrup (optional)

Directions

1. Place the riced cauliflower, almond milk, 2 tablespoons of olive oil, orange peel, almond extract, cinnamon, and salt in a medium saucepan.

2. Stir to incorporate and bring the mixture to a boil over medium-high heat, stirring often.

3. Remove from the heat and add 2 tablespoons of chopped walnuts and maple syrup (if desired).

4. Stir again and divide the porridge into bowls. To serve, sprinkle each bowl evenly with remaining 2 tablespoons of walnuts and olive oil.

Per Serving

calories: 381 | fat: 37.8g | protein: 5.2g | carbs: 10.9g | fiber: 4.0g | sodium: 228mg

Arugula and Fig Salad

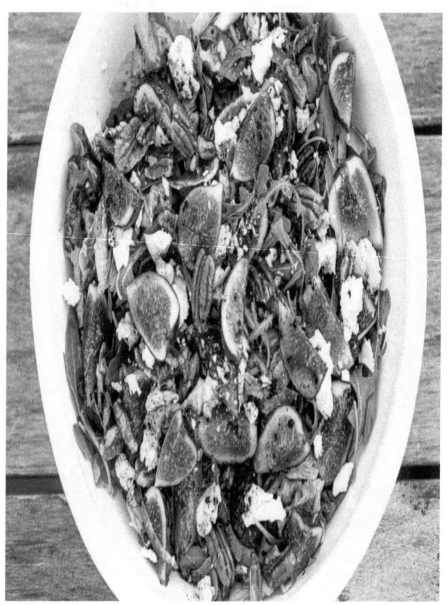

Prep time:

15 minutes | Cook time: 0 minutes | Serves 2

Ingredients

3 cups arugula

4 fresh, ripe figs (or 4 to 6 dried figs), stemmed and sliced

2 tablespoons olive oil

¼ cup lightly toasted pecan halves

2 tablespoons crumbled blue cheese

1 to 2 tablespoons balsamic glaze

Directions

1. Toss the arugula and figs with the olive oil in a large bowl until evenly coated.

2. Add the pecans and blue cheese to the bowl. Toss the salad lightly.

3. Drizzle with the balsamic glaze and serve immediately.

Per Serving

calories: 517 | fat: 36.2g | protein: 18.9g | carbs: 30.2g | fiber: 6.1g | sodium: 481mg

Mediterranean Greek Salad Wraps

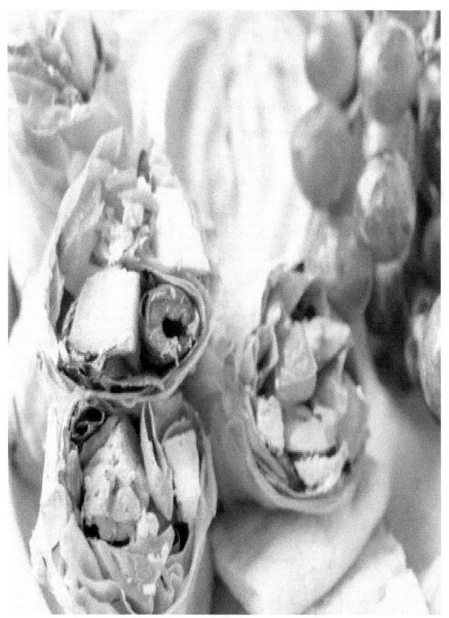

Prep time:

15 minutes | Cook time: 0 minutes | Serves 4

Ingredients

1½ cups seedless cucumber, peeled and chopped

1 cup chopped tomato

½ cup finely chopped fresh mint

¼ cup diced red onion

1 (2.25-ounce / 64-g) can sliced black olives, drained

2 tablespoons extra-virgin olive oil

1 tablespoon red wine vinegar

¼ teaspoon kosher salt

¼ teaspoon freshly ground black pepper

½ cup crumbled goat cheese

4 whole-wheat flatbread wraps or soft whole-wheat tortillas

Directions

1. In a large bowl, stir together the cucumber, tomato, mint, onion and olives.

2. In a small bowl, whisk together the oil, vinegar, salt, and pepper. Spread the dressing over the salad. Toss gently to combine.

3. On a clean work surface, lay the wraps. Divide the goat cheese evenly among the wraps. Scoop a quarter of the salad filling down the center of each wrap.

4. Fold up each wrap: Start by folding up the bottom, then fold one side over and fold the other side over the top. Repeat with the remaining wraps.

5. Serve immediately.

Per Serving

calories: 225 | fat: 12.0g | protein: 12.0g | carbs: 18.0g | fiber: 4.0g | sodium: 349mg

Rice and Blueberry Stuffed Sweet Potatoes

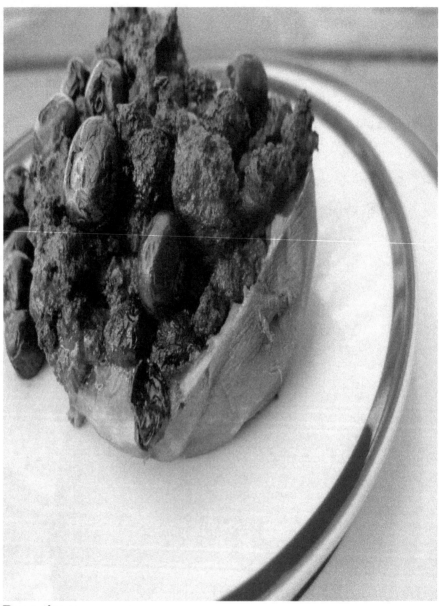

Prep time:

15 minutes | Cook time: 20 minutes | Serves 4

Ingredients

2 cups cooked wild rice

½ cup dried blueberries

½ cup chopped hazelnuts

½ cup shredded Swiss chard

1 teaspoon chopped fresh thyme

1 scallion, white and green parts, peeled and thinly sliced

Sea salt and freshly ground black pepper, to taste

4 sweet potatoes, baked in the skin until tender

Directions

1. Preheat the oven to 400°F (205°C).

2. Combine all the Ingredients, except for the sweet potatoes, in a large bowl. Stir to mix well.

3. Cut the top third of the sweet potato off length wire, then scoop most of the sweet potato flesh out.

4. Fill the potato with the wild rice mixture, then set the sweet potato on a greased baking sheet.

5. Bake in the preheated oven for 20 minutes or until the sweet potato skin is lightly charred.

6. Serve immediately.

Per Serving

calories: 393 | fat: 7.1g | protein: 10.2g | carbs: 76.9g | fiber: 10.0g | sodium: 93mg

Asparagus and Broccoli Primavera Farfalle

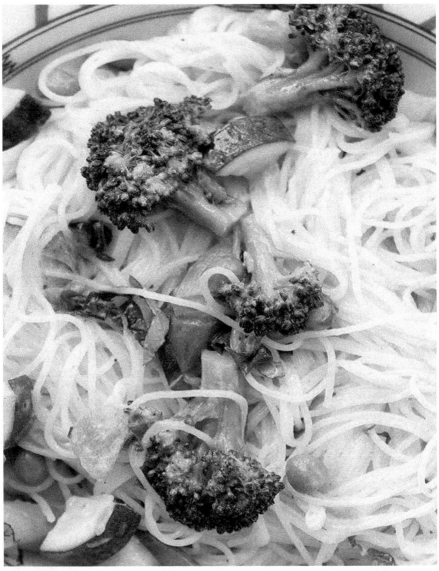

Prep time:

15 minutes | Cook time: 12 minutes | Serves 4

Ingredients

1 bunch asparagus, trimmed, cut into 1-inch pieces

2 cups broccoli florets

3 tablespoons olive oil

3 teaspoons salt

10 ounces (283 g) egg noodles

3 garlic cloves, minced

2½ cups vegetable stock

½ cup heavy cream

1 cup small tomatoes, halved

¼ cup chopped basil

½ cup grated Parmesan cheese

Directions

1. Pour 2 cups of water, add the noodles, 2 tablespoons of olive oil, garlic and salt. Place a trivet over the water. Combine asparagus, broccoli, remaining olive oil and salt in a bowl. Place the vegetables on the trivet.

2. Seal the lid and cook on Steam for 12 minutes on High. Do a quick release. Remove the vegetables to a plate. Stir the heavy cream and tomatoes in the pasta. Press Sauté and simmer the cream until desired consistency. Gently mix in the asparagus and broccoli. Garnish with basil and Parmesan, to serve.

Per Serving

calories: 544 | fat: 23.8g | protein: 18.5g | carbs: 66.1g | fiber: 6.0g | sodium: 2354mg

Lentils and Eggplant Curry

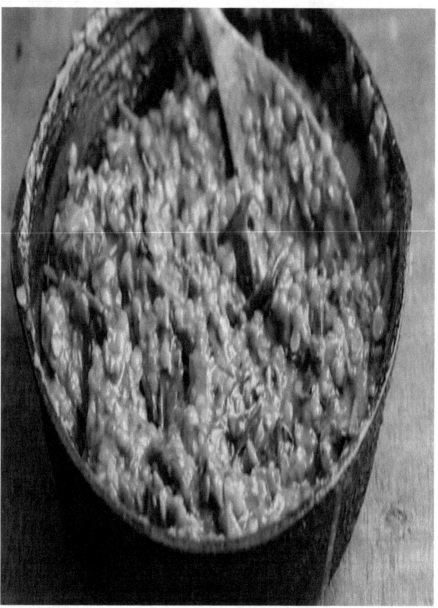

Prep time:

10 minutes | Cook time: 22 minutes | Serves 4

Ingredients

¾ cup lentils, soaked and rinsed

1 teaspoon olive oil

½ onion, chopped

4 garlic cloves, chopped

1 teaspoon ginger, chopped

1 hot green chili, chopped

¼ teaspoon turmeric

½ teaspoon ground cumin

2 tomatoes, chopped

1 cup eggplant, chopped

1 cup sweet potatoes, cubed

¾ teaspoon salt

2 cups water

1 cup baby spinach leaves

Cayenne and lemon/lime to taste

Pepper flakes (garnish)

Directions

1. Add the oil, garlic, ginger, chili and salt into the instant pot and Sauté for 3 minutes.

2. Stir in the tomatoes and all the spices. Cook for 5 minutes.

3. Add all the remaining Ingredients, except the spinach leaves and garnish.

4. Secure the lid and cook on Manual function for 12 minutes at High Pressure.

5. After the beep, release the pressure naturally and remove the lid.

6. Stir in the spinach leaves and let the pot simmer for 2 minutes on Sauté.

7. Garnish with the pepper flakes and serve warm.

Per Serving

calories: 88 | fat: 1.5g | protein: 3.4g | carbs: 17.4g | fiber: 3.3g | sodium: 470mg

Parmesan Stuffed Zucchini Boats

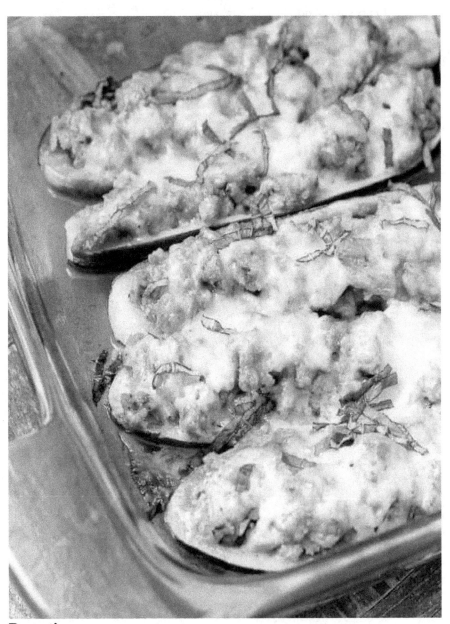

Prep time:

5 minutes | Cook time: 15 minutes | Serves 4

Ingredients

1 cup canned low-sodium chickpeas, drained and rinsed

1 cup no-sugar-added spaghetti sauce

2 zucchinis

¼ cup shredded Parmesan cheese

Directions

1. Preheat the oven to 425°F (220°C).

2. In a medium bowl, stir together the chickpeas and spaghetti sauce.

3. Cut the zucchini in half lengthwise and scrape a spoon gently down the length of each half to remove the seeds.

4. Fill each zucchini half with the chickpea sauce and top with one-quarter of the Parmesan cheese.

5. Place the zucchini halves on a baking sheet and roast in the oven for 15 minutes.

6. Transfer to a plate. Let rest for 5 minutes before serving.

Per Serving

calories: 139 | fat: 4.0g | protein: 8.0g | carbs: 20.0g | fiber: 5.0g | sodium: 344mg

Celery and Mustard Greens

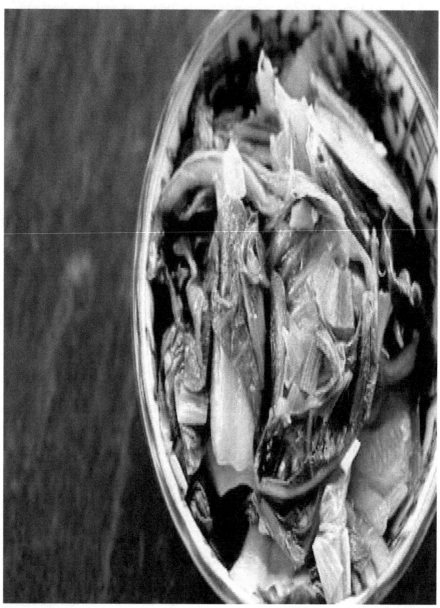

Prep time:

10 minutes | Cook time: 15 minutes | Serves 4

Ingredients

½ cup low-sodium vegetable broth

1 celery stalk, roughly chopped

½ sweet onion, chopped

½ large red bell pepper, thinly sliced

2 garlic cloves, minced

1 bunch mustard greens, roughly chopped

Directions

1. Pour the vegetable broth into a large cast iron pan and bring it to a simmer over medium heat.

2. Stir in the celery, onion, bell pepper, and garlic. Cook uncovered for about 3 to 5 minutes, or until the onion is softened.

3. Add the mustard greens to the pan and stir well. Cover, reduce the heat to low, and cook for an additional 10 minutes, or until the liquid is evaporated and the greens are wilted.

4. Remove from the heat and serve warm.

Per Serving (1 cup)

calories: 39 | fat: 0g | protein: 3.1g | carbs: 6.8g | fiber: 3.0g | sodium: 120mg

Zucchini Patties

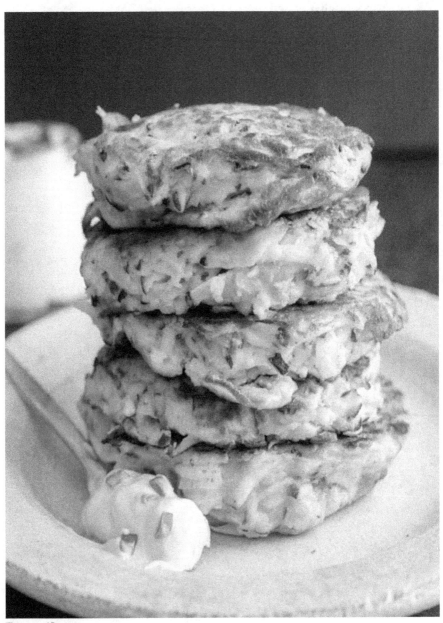

Prep time:

15 minutes | Cook time: 5 minutes | Serves 2

Ingredients

2 medium zucchinis, shredded

1 teaspoon salt, divided

2 eggs

2 tablespoons chickpea flour

1 tablespoon chopped fresh mint

1 scallion, chopped

2 tablespoons extra-virgin olive oil

Directions

1. Put the shredded zucchini in a fine-mesh strainer and season with ½ teaspoon of salt. Set aside.

2. Beat together the eggs, chickpea flour, mint, scallion, and remaining ½ teaspoon of salt in a medium bowl.

3. Squeeze the zucchini to drain as much liquid as possible. Add the zucchini to the egg mixture and stir until well incorporated.

4. Heat the olive oil in a large skillet over medium-high heat.

5. Drop the zucchini mixture by spoonfuls into the skillet. Gently flatten the zucchini with the back of a spatula.

6. Cook for 2 to 3 minutes or until golden brown. Flip and cook for an additional 2 minutes.

7. Remove from the heat and serve on a plate.

Per Serving

calories: 264 | fat: 20.0g | protein: 9.8g | carbs: 16.1g | fiber: 4.0g | sodium: 1780mg

Panko Grilled Chicken Patties

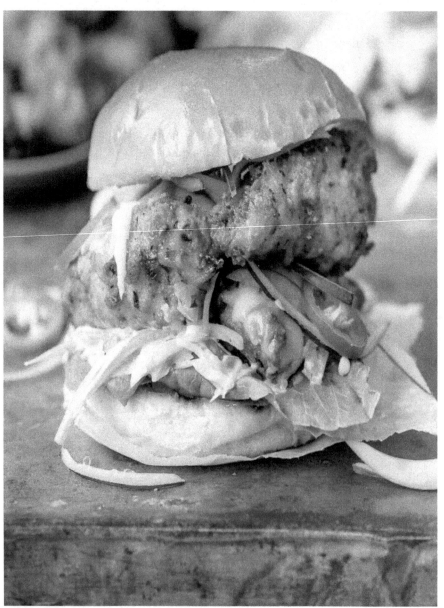

Prep time:

10 minutes | Cook time: 8 to 10 minutes | Serves 4

Ingredients

1 pound (454 g) ground chicken

3 tablespoons crumbled feta cheese

3 tablespoons finely chopped red pepper

¼ cup finely chopped red onion

3 tablespoons panko bread crumbs

1 garlic clove, minced

1 teaspoon chopped fresh oregano

¼ teaspoon salt

⅛ teaspoon freshly ground black pepper

Cooking spray

Directions

1. Mix together the ground chicken, feta cheese, red pepper, red onion, bread crumbs, garlic, oregano, salt, and black pepper in a large bowl, and stir to incorporate.

2. Divide the chicken mixture into 8 equal portions and form each portion into a patty with your hands.

3. Preheat a grill to medium-high heat and oil the grill grates with cooking spray.

4. Arrange the patties on the grill grates and grill each side for 4 to 5 minutes, or until the patties are cooked through.

5. Rest for 5 minutes before serving.

Per Serving

calories: 241 | fat: 13.5g | protein: 23.2g | carbs:6.7g | fiber: 1.1g | sodium: 321mg

Garlic Shrimp with Mushrooms

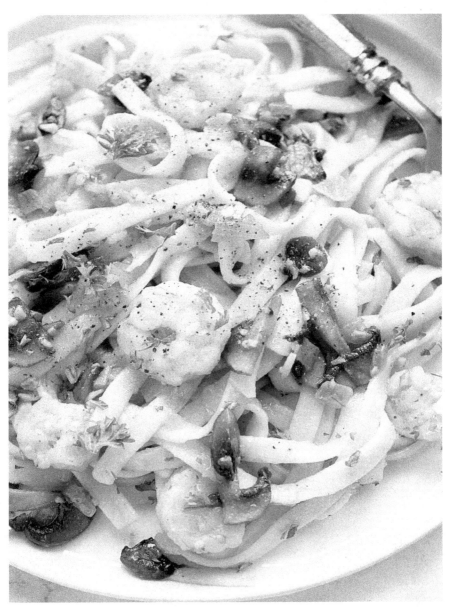

Prep time:

10 minutes | Cook time: 15 minutes | Serves 4

Ingredients

1 pound (454 g) fresh shrimp, peeled, deveined, and patted dry

1 teaspoon salt

1 cup extra-virgin olive oil

8 large garlic cloves, thinly sliced

4 ounces (113 g) sliced mushrooms (shiitake, baby bella, or button)

½ teaspoon red pepper flakes

¼ cup chopped fresh flat-leaf Italian parsley

Directions

1. In a bowl, season the shrimp with salt. Set aside.

2. Heat the olive oil in a large skillet over medium-low heat.

3. Add the garlic and cook for 3 to 4 minutes until fragrant, stirring occasionally.

4. Saut é the mushrooms for 5 minutes, or until they start to exude their juices.

5. Stir in the shrimp and sprinkle with red pepper flakes and saut é for 3 to 4 minutes more, or until the shrimp start to turn pink.

6. Remove the skillet from the heat and add the parsley. Stir to combine and serve warm.

Per Serving

calories: 619 | fat: 55.5g | protein: 24.1g | carbs: 3.7g | fiber: 0g | sodium: 735mg

Spicy Grilled Shrimp with Lemon Wedges

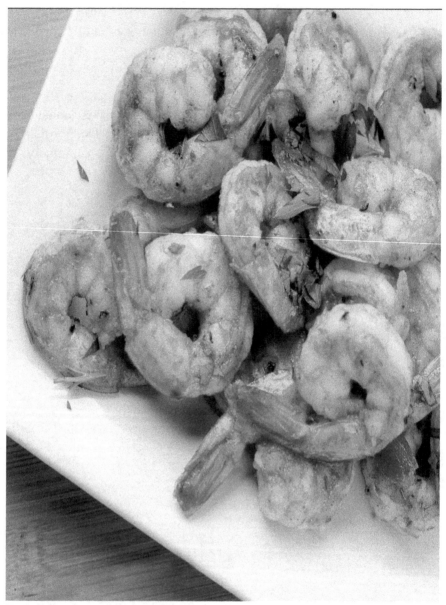

Prep time:

15 minutes | Cook time: 6 minutes | Serves 6

Ingredients

1 large clove garlic, crushed

1 teaspoon coarse salt

1 teaspoon paprika

½ teaspoon cayenne pepper

2 teaspoons lemon juice

2tablespoons plus 1 teaspoon olive oil, divided

2 pounds (907 g) large shrimp, peeled and deveined

8 wedges lemon, for garnish

Directions

1. Preheat the grill to medium heat.

2. Stir together the garlic, salt, paprika, cayenne pepper, lemon juice, and 2 tablespoons of olive oil in a small bowl until a paste forms. Add the shrimp and toss until well coated.

3. Grease the grill grates lightly with remaining 1 teaspoon of olive oil.

4. Grill the shrimp for 4 to 6 minutes, flipping the shrimp halfway through, or until the shrimp is totally pink and opaque.

5. Garnish the shrimp with lemon wedges and serve hot.

Per Serving

calories: 163 | fat: 5.8g | protein: 25.2g | carbs: 2.8g | fiber: 0.4g | sodium: 585mg

Rosemary Salmon with Feta Cheese

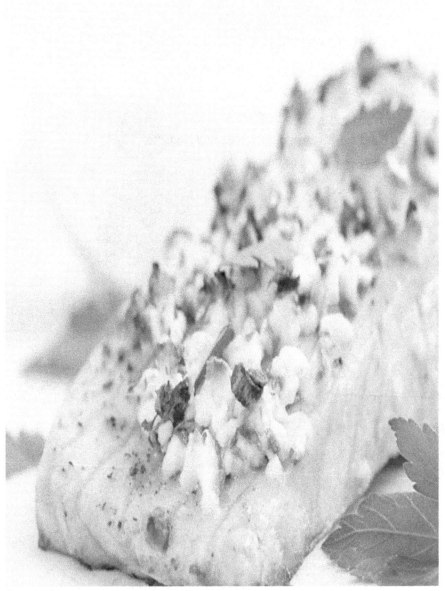

Prep time:

5 minutes | Cook time: 3 minutes | Serves 6

Ingredients

1½ pounds (680 g) salmon fillets

1½ cups water

¼ cup olive oil

1½ garlic cloves, minced

1½ tablespoons feta cheese, crumbled

½ teaspoon dried oregano

3 tablespoons fresh lemon juice

Salt and freshly ground black pepper, to taste

3 fresh rosemary sprigs

3 lemon slices

Directions

1. Take a large bowl and add the garlic, feta cheese, salt, pepper, lemon juice, and oregano. Whisk well all the Ingredients.

2. Add the water to the Instant pot then place the steamer trivet in it.

3. Arrange the salmon fillets over the trivet in a single layer.

4. Pour the cheese mixture over these fillets.

5. Place a lemon slice and a rosemary sprig over each fillet.

6. Secure the lid.

7. Select the Steam function on your cooker and set 3 minutes cooking time.

8. After it is done, carefully do a Quick release. Remove the lid.

9. Serve hot.

Per Serving

calories: 229 | fat: 14.0g | protein: 23.4g | carbs: 1.3g | fiber: 0.2g | sodium: 88mg

Mint Banana Chocolate Sorbet

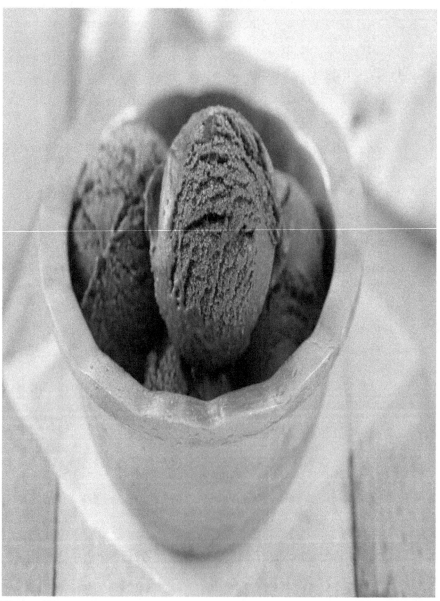

Prep time:

4 hours 5 minutes | Cook time: 0 minutes | Serves 1

Ingredients

1 frozen banana

1 tablespoon almond butter

2 tablespoons minced fresh mint

2 to 3 tablespoons dark chocolate chips (60% cocoa or higher)

2 to 3 tablespoons goji (optional)

Directions

1. Put the banana, butter, and mint in a food processor. Pulse to purée until creamy and smooth.

2. Add the chocolate and goji, then pulse for several more times to combine well.

3. Pour the mixture in a bowl or a ramekin, then freeze for at least 4 hours before serving chilled.

Per Serving

calories: 213 | fat: 9.8g | protein: 3.1g | carbs: 2.9g | fiber: 4.0g | sodium: 155mg

Apple and Berries Ambrosia

Prep time:

15 minutes | Cook time: 0 minutes | Serves 4

Ingredients

2 cups unsweetened coconut milk, chilled

2 tablespoons raw honey

1 apple, peeled, cored, and chopped

2 cups fresh raspberries

2 cups fresh blueberries

Directions

1. Spoon the chilled milk in a large bowl, then mix in the honey. Stir to mix well.

2. Then mix in the remaining Ingredients. Stir to coat the fruits well and serve immediately.

Per Serving

calories: 386 | fat: 21.1g | protein: 4.2g | carbs: 45.9g | fiber: 11.0g | sodium: 16mg

Italian Dressing

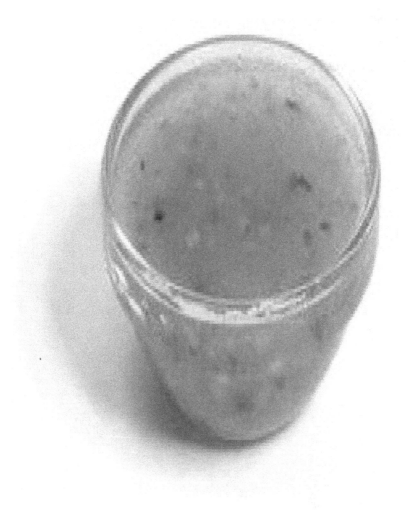

Prep time:

5 minutes | Cook time: 0 minutes | Serves 12

Ingredients

½ cup extra-virgin olive oil

¼ cup red wine vinegar

1 teaspoon dried Italian seasoning

1 teaspoon Dijon mustard

¼ teaspoon salt

¼ teaspoon freshly ground black pepper

1 garlic clove, minced

Directions

1. Place all the Ingredients in a mason jar and cover. Shake vigorously for 1 minute until completely mixed.

2. Store in the refrigerator for up to 1 week.

Per Serving (1 tablespoon)

calories: 80 | fat: 8.6g | protein: 0g | carbs: 0g | fiber: 0g | sodium: 51mg

Hot Pepper Sauce

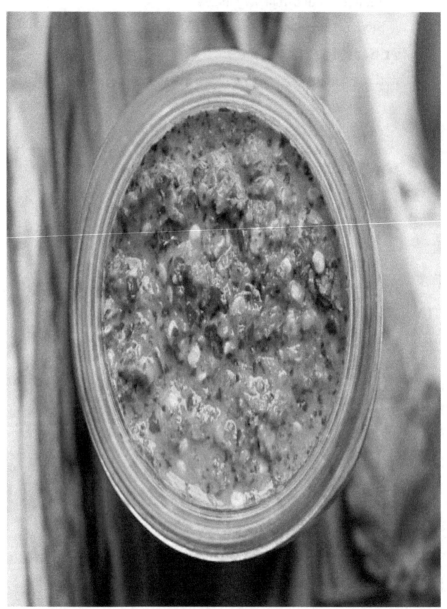

Prep time:

10 minutes | Cook time: 20 minutes | Makes 4 cups

Ingredients

1 red hot fresh chiles, deseeded

2 dried chiles

2 garlic cloves, peeled

½ small yellow onion, roughly chopped

2 cups water

2 cups white vinegar

Directions

1. Place all the Ingredients except the vinegar in a medium saucepan over medium heat. Allow to simmer for 20 minutes until softened.

2. Transfer the mixture to a food processor or blender. Stir in the vinegar and pulse until very smooth.

3. Serve immediately or transfer to a sealed container and refrigerate for up to 3 months.

Per Serving (2 tablespoons)

calories: 20 | fat: 1.2g | protein: 0.6g | carbs: 4.4g | fiber: 0.6g | sodium: 12mg

No Cook Overnight Oats

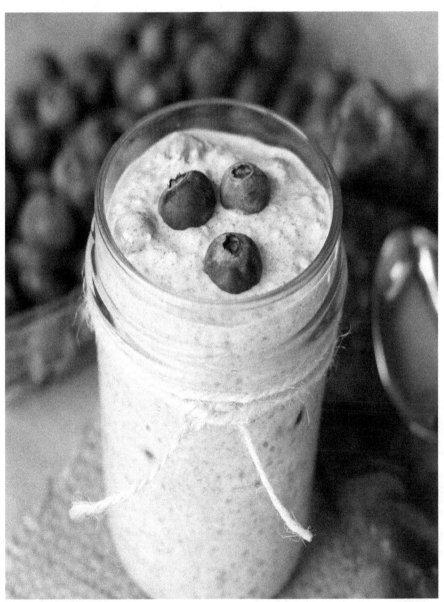

Preparation time:

5 minutes Cooking time: 0 minutes Servings: 1

Ingredients:

- 1 ½ c. low-fat milk
- 5 whole almond pieces 1 tsp. chia seeds
- 2 tbsps. Oats
- 1 tsp. sunflower seeds 1 tbsp. Craisins

Directions:

1. In a jar or mason bottle with a cap, mix all Ingredients. Refrigerate overnight. Enjoy for breakfast.

Nutrition: Calories: 271 Fat:9.8 g Carbs:35.4 g Protein:16.7 g Sugars:9 Sodium:103 mg

Spinach Muffins

Preparation time:

10 minutes Cooking time: 30 minutes Servings: 6

Ingredients:

- 6 eggs
- ½ cup non-fat milk
- cup low-fat cheese, crumbled 4 ounces spinach
- ½ cup roasted red pepper, chopped 2 ounces prosciutto, chopped Cooking spray

Directions:

1. Mix the eggs with the milk, cheese, spinach, red pepper, and prosciutto in a bowl. Greas a muffin tray with cooking spray, divide the muffin mix, introduce in the oven, and bake at 350 degrees F within 30 minutes. Divide between plates and serve for breakfast.

Nutrition: Calories: 112 Carbs: 19g Fat: 3g Protein: 2g

Sodium: 274 mg

Buckwheat Pancakes with Vanilla Almond Milk

Preparation time:

10 minutes Cooking time: 10 minutes Servings: 1

Ingredients:

- ½ c. unsweetened vanilla almond milk 2-4 packets natural sweetener
- 1/8 tsp salt
- ½ cup buckwheat flour
- ½ tsp. double-acting baking powder

Directions:

1. Prepare a nonstick pancake griddle and spray with the cooking spray, place over medium heat. Whisk the buckwheat flour, salt, baking powder, and stevia in a small bowl and stir in the almond milk after.

2. Onto the pan, scoop a large spoonful of batter, cook until bubbles no longer pop on the surface and the entire surface looks dry and (2-4 minutes). Flip and cook for another 2-4 minutes. Repeat with all the remaining batter.

Nutrition: Calories: 240 Fat:4.5 g Carbs:2 g Protein:11 g Sugars:17 g Sodium:38 mg

Salsa Chicken

Preparation time:

10 minutes Cooking time: 25 minutes Servings: 4

Ingredients:

- 1 cup mild salsa, no-salt-added
- ½ teaspoon cumin, ground Black pepper to the taste
- tablespoon chipotle paste
- 1-pound chicken thighs, skinless and boneless 2 cups corn
- Juice of 1 lime
- tablespoon olive oil
- tablespoons cilantro, chopped 1 cup cherry tomatoes, halved
- 1 small avocado, pitted, peeled, and cubed

Directions:

1. In a pot, combine the salsa with the cumin, black pepper, chipotle paste, chicken thighs, and corn, toss, bring to a simmer and cook over medium heat for 25 minutes. Add lime juice, oil, cherry tomatoes, and avocado, toss, divide into bowls and serve for lunch. Enjoy!

Nutrition: Calories 269 Fat 6g

Fiber 9g Carbs 18g Protein 7g

Sodium 500 mg

Italian Stuffed Portobello Mushroom Burgers

Preparation time:

15 minutes Cooking time: 25 minutes Servings: 4

Ingredients:

- 1 tablespoon olive oil
- 4 large portobello mushrooms, washed and dried
- ½ yellow onion, peeled and diced 4 garlic cloves, peeled and minced 1 can cannellini beans, drained
- ½ cup fresh basil leaves, torn
- ½ cup panko bread crumbs 1/8 teaspoon kosher or sea salt
- ¼ teaspoon ground black pepper
- 1 cup lower-sodium marinara, divided
- ½ cup shredded mozzarella cheese 4 whole-wheat buns, toasted
- cup fresh arugula

Directions:

1. Heat-up the olive oil in a large skillet to medium-high heat. Sear the mushrooms for 4 to 5 minutes per side, until slightly soft. Place on a baking sheet. Preheat the oven to a low broil.

2. Put the onion in the skillet and cook for 4 to 5 minutes, until slightly soft. Mix in the garlic then cooks within 30 to 60 seconds. Move the onions plus garlic to a bowl. Add the cannellini beans and smash with the back of a fork to form a chunky paste. Stir in the basil, bread crumbs, salt, and black pepper and half of the marinara. Cook for 5 minutes.

3. Remove the bean mixture from the stove and divide among the mushroom caps. Spoon the remaining marinara over the stuffed mushrooms and top each with the mozzarella cheese. Broil within 3 to 4 minutes, until the cheese is melted and bubbly. Transfer the burgers to the toasted whole-wheat buns and top with the arugula.

Nutrition: Calories: 407 Fat: 9g Sodium: 575mg

Carbohydrate: 63g Protein: 25g

Aromatic Whole Grain Spaghetti

Preparation time:

15 minutes Cooking time: 10 minutes Servings: 2

Ingredients:

- 1 teaspoon dried basil
- ¼ cup of soy milk
- 6 oz whole-grain spaghetti 2 cups of water
- teaspoon ground nutmeg

Directions:

1. Bring the water to boil, add spaghetti, and cook them for 8-10 minutes. Meanwhile, bring the soy milk to boil. Drain the cooked spaghetti and mix them up with soy milk, ground nutmeg, and dried basil. Stir the meal well.

Nutrition: Calories 128 Protein 5.6g

Carbohydrates 25g Fat 1.4g

Sodium 25mg

No-Mayo Potato Salad

Preparation time:

15 minutes Cooking time: 20 minutes Servings: 8

Ingredients:

- Red potatoes – 3 pounds Extra virgin olive oil - .5 cup
- White wine vinegar, divided – 5 tablespoons
- Dijon mustard – 2 teaspoons Red onion, sliced – 1 cup
- Black pepper, ground - .5 teaspoon
- Basil, fresh, chopped – 2 tablespoons
- Dill weed, fresh, chopped – 2 tablespoons Parsley, fresh, chopped – 2 tablespoons

Directions:

1. Add the red potatoes to a large pot and cover them with water until the water level is two inches above the potatoes. Put the pot on high heat, then boil potatoes until they are tender when poked with a fork, about fifteen to twenty minutes. Drain off the water.

2. Let the potatoes to cool until they can easily be handled but are still warm, then cut it in half and put them in a large bowl. Stir in three tablespoons of the white wine vinegar, giving the potatoes a good stir so that they can evenly absorb the vinegar.

3. Mix the rest of two tablespoons of vinegar, extra virgin olive oil, Dijon mustard, and black pepper in a small bowl. Add this mixture to the potatoes and give them a good toss to thoroughly coat the potatoes.

4. Toss in the red onion and minced herbs. Serve at room temperature or chilled. Serve immediately or store in the fridge for up to four days.

Nutrition: Calories: 144

Carbs: 19g Fat: 7g Protein: 2g Sodium: 46mg

Chili Broccoli

Preparation time:

10 minutes Cooking time: 30 minutes Servings: 4

Ingredients:

- tablespoons olive oil 1-pound broccoli florets 2 garlic cloves, minced
- 2 tablespoons chili sauce 1 tablespoon lemon juice A pinch of black pepper
- 2 tablespoons cilantro, chopped

Directions:

1. In a baking pan, combine the broccoli with the oil, garlic, and the other, toss a bit, and bake at 400 degrees F for 30 minutes. Divide the mix between plates and serve as a side dish.

Nutrition: Calories 103 Protein 3.4g

Carbohydrates 8.3gz 7.4g fat

3g fiber

Sodium 229mg Potassium 383mg

Easy Carrots Mix

Preparation time:

10 minutes Cooking time: 40 minutes Servings: 6

Ingredients:

- 15 carrots, halved lengthwise 2 tablespoons coconut sugar
- ¼ cup olive oil
- ½ teaspoon rosemary, dried
- ½ teaspoon garlic powder A pinch of black pepper

Directions:

1. In a bowl, combine the carrots with the sugar, oil, rosemary, garlic powder, and black pepper, toss well, spread on a lined baking sheet, introduce in the oven and bake at 400 degrees F for 40 minutes. Serve.

Nutrition: Calories: 60 Carbs: 9g Fat: 0g Protein: 2g

Sodium: 0 mg

Chickpeas and Curried Veggies

Preparation time:

15 minutes Cooking time: 4 hours Servings: 2

Ingredients:

- ½ tbsp. Canola Oil 2 sliced Celery Ribs
- 1/8 tsp. Cayenne Pepper
- ¼ cup Water
- sliced Carrots
- 2 sliced red Potatoes (sliced)
- ½ tbsp. Curry Powder
- ½ cup of Coconut Milk (light)
- ¼ cup drained Chickpeas (low sodium) Chopped Cilantro
- ¼ cup Yogurt (low fat)

Directions:

1. Sauté potatoes for 5 mins in oil. Add the carrots, celery, and onion. Sauté for 5 more mins. Sprinkle on the curry powder and cayenne pepper. Stir well to combine.

2. In a slow cooker, pour water and coconut milk. Add in the potatoes. Cook on "low" for 3 hrs. Add chickpeas and cook for 30 more mins. Serve in bowls along with the yogurt and cilantro garnish.

Nutrition: Calories 271

Fats 11 g

Sodium 207 mg

Carbohydrates 39 g

Protein 7 g

Loaded Baked Sweet Potatoes

Preparation time:

15 minutes Cooking time: 20 minutes Servings: 4

Ingredients:

- 4 sweet potatoes
- ½ cup nonfat or low-fat plain Greek yogurt Freshly ground black pepper
- 1 teaspoon olive oil
- 1 red bell pepper, cored and diced
- ½ red onion, diced
- 1 teaspoon ground cumin
- 1 (15-ounce) can chickpeas, drained and rinsed

Directions:

1. Prick the potatoes using a fork and cook on your microwave's potato setting until potatoes are soft and cooked through, about 8 to 10 minutes for 4 potatoes. If you don't have a microwave, bake at 400°F for about 45 minutes.

2. Combine the yogurt and black pepper in a small bowl and mix well. Heat the oil in a medium pot over medium heat. Add bell pepper, onion, cumin, and additional black pepper to taste.

3. Add the chickpeas, stir to combine, and heat through about 5 minutes. Slice the potatoes lengthwise down the middle and top each half with a portion of the bean mixture followed by 1 to 2 tablespoons of the yogurt. Serve immediately.

Nutrition: Calories: 264 Fat: 2g Sodium: 124mg

Carbohydrate: 51g

Protein: 11g

Garlic and Lemon Soup

Preparation time:

15 minutes Cooking time: 0 minutes Servings: 3

Ingredients:

- avocado, pitted and chopped 1 cucumber, chopped
- bunches spinach
- 1 ½ cups watermelon, chopped
- bunch cilantro, roughly chopped Juice from 2 lemons
- ½ cup coconut aminos
- ½ cup lime juice

Directions:

1. Add cucumber, avocado to your blender, and pulse well. Add cilantro, spinach, and watermelon and blend. Add lemon, lime juice, and coconut amino. Pulse a few more times. Transfer to a soup bowl and enjoy!

Nutrition: Calories: 100 Fat: 7g

Carbohydrates: 6g Protein: 3g Sodium: 0 mg

Tabouleh Salad

Preparation time:

15 minutes Cooking time: 0 minutes Servings: 4

Ingredients:

- 2/3 cup dry couscous 1 cup boiling water
- 1 small ripe tomato, diced
- 1 small green bell pepper, diced 1 shallot, finely diced
- 1/3 cup chopped fresh parsley
- clove garlic, minced Juice of 1 fresh lemon 1 tablespoon olive oil
- 1/2 teaspoon freshly ground black pepper

Directions:

1. Mix the dry couscous into a small bowl. Mix in the boiling water, cover, and set aside within 5 minutes. Place the tomato, green pepper, shallot, and parsley into a salad bowl.

2. Mix the garlic, lemon juice, oil, and pepper in a small mixing bowl. Put the cooked couscous in the salad bowl. Put the dressing over the top and stir well to combine. Serve immediately.

Nutrition: Calories: 120

Fat: 3 g

Protein: 3 g

Sodium: 6 mg

Fiber: 1 g

Carbohydrates: 20 g

Sugar: 1 g

Turkey Wrap

Preparation time:

15 minutes Cooking time: 0 minutes Servings: 2

Ingredients:

- 2 slices of low-fat Turkey breast (deli-style) 4 tablespoon non-fat cream cheese
- ½ cup lettuce leaves
- ½ cup carrots, slice into a stick
- 2 Homemade wraps or store-bought whole-wheat tortilla wrap

Directions:

1. Prepare all the Ingredients. Spread 2 tablespoons of non-fat cream cheese on each wrap. Arrange lettuce leaves, then add a slice of turkey breast; a slice of carrots stick on top. Roll and cut into half. Serve and enjoy!

Nutrition: Calories 224

Carbohydrates 35g Protein 10.3g

Fat 3.8g

Sodium 293mg

Karen's Apple Kugel

Preparation time:

15 minutes Cooking time: 25 minutes Servings: 8

Ingredients:

- sheets unsalted matzo 2 cups of water
- tart green apples
- 1 tablespoon freshly squeezed lemon juice 3 tablespoons unsalted butter, melted
- 1/4 cup brown sugar
- 1/2 cup seedless raisins 3 egg whites
- 11/2 teaspoons ground cinnamon

Directions:

1. Preheat oven to 400°F. Take out an 8" × 11" baking dish and set aside. Place the matzo in an 8-inch square baking pan. Pour the water into the pan and set aside to rehydrate.

2. Peel apples, core, and cut into quarters. Cut each quarter crosswise into thirds and then lengthwise into slices no more than 1/4 inch thick. Transfer apples to a mixing bowl.

3. Check on the matzo. When soft, drain the matzo and squeeze out excess water. Place matzo into the mixing bowl. Put the rest of the fixing and stir well to combine.

4. Pour mixture into the 8" × 11" baking dish. Bake within 25 minutes. Remove from the oven. Set on a wire rack to cool. Cut into portions and serve warm or cool.

Nutrition: Calories: 181

Fat: 4 g

Protein: 3 g

Sodium: 24 mg

Fiber: 2 g

Carbohydrates: 34 g

Sugar: 21 g

Peach Cobbler

Preparation time:

15 minutes Cooking time: 25 minutes Servings: 8

Ingredients:

- 6 ripe peaches, peeled and sliced 3 tablespoons sugar

- Juice of 1 fresh lemon

- 11/4 cups unbleached all-purpose flour 1/2 cup white whole-wheat flour

- 2/3 cup sugar

- 1 teaspoon sodium-free baking powder

- 4 tablespoons unsalted butter, melted and cooled 1 egg white

- 1/2 cup low-fat milk

- 1 tablespoon pure vanilla extract

Directions:

1. Preheat oven to 425°F. Take out a 9" × 13" baking dish and set aside. Put the sliced peaches into a mixing bowl, put sugar plus lemon juice, and toss well to coat. Transfer to the baking dish. Set aside.

2. Mix the flours, sugar, plus baking powder into a mixing bowl. Add the melted butter, egg white, milk, and vanilla and stir well to combine. Scoop batter over sliced peaches.

3. Put baking dish on middle rack in the oven, then bake for 25 minutes. Remove dish from oven and place on a wire rack to cool. Serve warm or cool.

Nutrition: Calories: 273

Fat: 6 g

Protein: 5 g

Sodium: 15 mg

Fiber: 3 g

Carbohydrates: 50 g

Sugar: 28 g

Triple-Green Pasta with Cheese

Prep time:

5 minutes | Cook time: 14 to 16 minutes | Serves 4

Ingredients

8 ounces (227 g) uncooked penne

1 tablespoon extra-virgin olive oil

2 garlic cloves, minced

¼ teaspoon crushed red pepper

2 cups chopped fresh flat-leaf parsley, including stems

5 cups loosely packed baby spinach

¼ teaspoon ground nutmeg

¼ teaspoon kosher salt

¼ teaspoon freshly ground black pepper

⅓ cup Castelvetrano olives, pitted and sliced

⅓ cup grated Parmesan cheese

Direction

1. In a large stockpot of salted water, cook the pasta for about 8 to 10 minutes. Drain the pasta and reserve ¼ cup of the cooking liquid.

2. Meanwhile, heat the olive oil in a large skillet over medium heat. Add the garlic and red pepper and cook for 30 seconds, stirring constantly.

3. Add the parsley and cook for 1 minute, stirring constantly. Add the spinach, nutmeg, salt, and pepper, and cook for 3 minutes, stirring occasionally, or until the spinach is wilted.

4. Add the cooked pasta and the reserved ¼ cup cooking liquid to the skillet. Stir in the olives and cook for about 2 minutes, or until most of the pasta water has been absorbed.

5. Remove from the heat and stir in the cheese before serving.

Per Serving

Calories: 262 | fat: 4.0g | protein: 15.0g | carbs: 51.0g | fiber: 13.0g | sodium: 1180mg

Alphabetical Index

T

Z

CPSIA information can be obtained
at www.ICGtesting.com
Printed in the USA
BVHW090116240521
607867BV00003B/938

9 781802 839036